The Self-Improvement Manual for Mental Well-Being:

How to Overcome Mental Imbalance

By

Dr. Micah K. Trump

Copyright © by Dr. Micah K. Trump 2022. All rights reserved.

Before this document is reproduced in any way, the publisher's permission must be given. Therefore, the contents within cannot neither be stored electronically, transferred, or isolated in a database.

No part of the document can be copied, scanned, retained, without approval from the creator.

TABLE OF CONTENTS

INTRODUCTION

Mental illnesses are among the most common health issues in the United States and throughout the globe. One out of every five Americans suffers from a mental illness. At some time in their life, more than half of all individuals will be diagnosed with a mental ailment or disorder. Unfortunately, mental health difficulties are developing on a daily basis and threaten to increase the number of cases in the next years, necessitating the need for a major mental awareness campaign.

Mental health awareness is a worldwide movement to eliminate the stigma associated with mental illness and mental health difficulties.

"The self-improvement manual for mental wellbeing" is a genuine effort

that seeks to strengthen the fight against mental health disorders and other related cases. Often people find solutions to their problems from two or more reading experiences (s); such an effort to provide solutions to one's mental health has been well researched and included in this manual for readers to not just read but also implement and find solutions to their mental instability. Not just causes of mental instability but also solutions have been included in this very book. Doubting your mental stability? **Then let this book be the one for you!**
Do have a wonderful reading experience.

Chapter 1
Mental illness is real; let's retain our sanity.

Definition of Mental Health?

Mental health is the entire well-being of how you think and manage your thoughts and conduct. Sometimes individuals encounter a major impairment in their mental functioning. A mental illness may be present when patterns or changes in thinking, feeling, or behavior create discomfort or undermine a person's capacity to function.

Your mental health; your psychological, emotional, and social well-being affects every part of your life.

Having a good mental health helps you to successfully cope with the everyday demands of life, interact well with others, make healthy choices and enjoy life to its fullest.
But occasionally, difficulties with mental diseases and addiction(s) may make it feel like obtaining a healthy mental state is unattainable.
Maintaining your mental health is crucial to living a happy, healthy life.
But regrettably, millions of individuals deal with mental diseases that leave them feeling hopeless, powerless, and alone.
Many resort to drugs and alcohol to ease this anguish and deal with the mental disorders they suffer.
It is very easy to feel overwhelmed these days.

With everything going on,
it's sort of challenging not to get
inundated by the sheer amount of
everything going on around the globe.
And our collective mental health is
hurting.
For instance, we had/have the Covid-
19 epidemic (or is it endemic), we
have politicians pulling us apart in the
name of togetherness, and we have a
never-ending sensation that the new
normal won't ever go back to the old
normal.
With all this lack of stability, it's no
surprise that most individuals feel a
heavy weight on their shoulders as
the burden of the unknown weighs
heavily on most of us. Especially at
work.

Maintaining a healthy mind is particularly crucial since a negative state of mind tends to generate brain-threatening sickness.

Mental disease, sometimes termed mental health disorders, refers to a broad spectrum of mental health issues - illnesses that impact your emotions, thinking, and conduct. Examples of mental illness include depression, anxiety disorders, schizophrenia, eating problems, and addictive habits.

Many individuals suffer mental health difficulties from time to time. But a mental health problem becomes a mental disease when recurring indications and symptoms cause regular stress and damage your capacity to perform.

A mental illness may make you unpleasant and can create issues in your everyday life, such as in school or work or in relationships

Examples of signs and symptoms include:
• Feeling sad or depressed
• Confused thinking or impaired ability to focus
• Excessive concerns or anxieties, or excessive emotions of guilt
• Extreme mood fluctuations of highs and lows
• Withdrawal from friends and activities
• Significant weariness, poor energy, or trouble sleeping
• Detachment from reality (delusions), paranoia, or hallucinations

• Inability to deal with everyday challenges or stress
• Trouble understanding and connecting to circumstances and to people
• Problems with alcohol or drug usage
• Major changes in dietary habits
• Sex desire alters
• Suicidal thoughts
Sometimes signs of a mental health illness show as physical concerns, such as stomach discomfort, back pain, headaches, or other inexplicable aches and pains.

Certain variables may raise your chance of getting a mental disease, including:
• A history of mental illness in blood-related, such as a parent or sibling

• Stressful life conditions, such as financial issues, a loved one's death, or a divorce
• A continuous (chronic) medical condition, such as diabetes
• Brain damage as a consequence of a catastrophic incident (traumatic brain injury), such as a forceful hit to the head
• Traumatic events, such as military combat or assault
• Use of alcohol or recreational drugs
Mental illness is frequent. About 1 in 5 individuals has a mental ailment in any given year.

The mental disease may begin at any age, from infancy to later adult years, although most instances begin earlier in life.

The impacts of mental disease might be brief or long-term.

You also may have more than one mental health problem at the same time.

For example, you may have depression plus a drug use problem. Mental disease is a primary cause of impairment. Untreated mental illness may cause significant emotional, behavioral and physical health difficulties. Complications often associated with mental disorders include:

• Unhappiness and diminished pleasure of life
• Family tensions
• Relationship troubles
• Social isolation
• Poverty and homelessness
• Self-injury and harm to others, including suicide or murder

• Weakened immune system, thus your body has a hard time rejecting infections

Benefits of a Good State of Mind. Just as physical fitness helps our body to remain strong, mental fitness enables us to develop and keep a condition of excellent mental health. When we are mentally well, we like our lives and surroundings, and the people in it. We may be creative, learn, try new things, and take chances. We are better equipped to deal with challenging moments in our personal and professional life.
We experience the anguish and fury that may come with the death of a loved one, a job loss or marital troubles, and other tough situations.

Although with time, we are able to move on and enjoy our lives once more.

Nurturing our mental health may also help us battle or avoid the mental health difficulties that are occasionally connected with a chronic physical condition. In rare situations, it may prevent the beginning or return of a medical or mental disorder. Managing stress correctly, for instance, may have a good influence on heart disease.

Chances are, you are already taking efforts to support your mental health, as well as your physical health you simply may not recognize it.

Below are some of the advantages of healthy mental health.

The Ability to Cope With The Ups and Downs of Life

When mental and emotional states are at the top levels, the obstacles of life might be simpler to conquer.
Where alcohol/drugs, solitude, tantrums, or fighting may have been taken to handle marital disagreements, financial troubles, job obstacles, and other life issues a stable mental state may enable healthy coping techniques.

A Positive Self-Image

Mental health closely links with personal thoughts about oneself. Overall mental well-being has a factor in your self-esteem. Confidence may frequently be a strong sign of a healthy mental condition.

A person whose mental health is thriving is more inclined to concentrate on the good in oneself. They will concentrate on these attributes, and will typically have aspirations that seek a healthy, happy existence.

Healthier Relationships

If your mental health is in excellent shape, you could be better capable of offering your friends and family quality time, love, and support. When you're not in emotional discomfort, it might be simpler to show up and support the people you care about.

Better Productivity

Dealing with depression or other mental health conditions might impair your productivity levels. If you feel mentally strong, it's more probable that you will be able to perform more effectively and deliver better quality work.

Higher Quality of Life

When mental well-being flourishes, your quality of life may improve. This may allow possibilities for increased engagement in community development. For example, you may begin helping in soup kitchens, food drives, shelters, etc.

You could also take up new activities, make new friends, and go to new cities.

Other advantages of strong mental health include :

1. Anxiety Reduction

There is several ways an anxiety illness might damage your health. Anxiety simply implies you are under continual tension as if you are being threatened. This may create numerous sorts of issues.

DIGESTIVE PROBLEMS.

One of the early difficulties induced by an anxiety illness is digestive problems, such as nausea, stomach cramps, and diarrhoea. You may reduce your appetite, leading you to lose weight. An anxiety problem may aggravate irritable bowel syndrome and Cohn's disease. Ulcers were originally considered to be caused by excessive stomach acid from stress, but have now been discovered to be caused by bacteria. However, prolonged worry may also damage your immune system, making you more prone to ulcers.

NEUROLOGICAL PROBLEMS.

When you have an anxiety problem, your sympathetic nervous system is working overtime. Your sympathetic nervous system, or SNS, is known as the "fight or flight" system, which is triggered by threats. It is designed to perform briefly, to get you out of difficulty, but when it's operating all the time, it creates health concerns. Certain biological tasks are the duty of the SNS, while others are the responsibility of the counteracting system, the parasympathetic nervous system, or PNS. When the SNS is underactive, you have greater problems resting and recuperating from accidents and diseases.

You may also have a lot more muscular tension, leading to headaches and back and joint discomfort.

CARDIOVASCULAR PROBLEMS.

Most individuals are now aware that stress is detrimental to your cardiovascular system. When you're stressed—and when you're nervous, you're typically stressed—your heart rate and blood pressure rise. Eventually, your blood arteries get stiffer, leading to a larger risk of heart attack and stroke.

RELATIONSHIPS

As social animals, having excellent connections is vital to happiness. Unfortunately, anxiety problems are often hard on relationships. Since nervousness reduces your readiness to attempt new things, it limits what you're willing to do with your pals. It may even impede your desire to meet new people and create friends. Ironically, the premium we put on social approval also causes social anxiety. The stakes simply seem too high for some individuals to risk rejection. Instead, they become socially isolated, and much more worried. Anxiety disorders may damage relationships in other ways too.

For example, if you have PTSD, you could become short-tempered and domineering, becoming irrationally upset with those you care about. This might alienate you or possibly lead to legal difficulties.
The repercussions of anxiety disorder are practically limitless. It is thus a necessity to keep our mental health under check!

2. Increased self-esteem.
What is self-esteem? At its most basic definition, self-esteem is how one regards oneself. It's a judgment that we impose on ourselves. Self-esteem has a direct relationship to our mental health and our quality of life.

Low self-esteem relates to feelings of despair and anxiety, as well as making bad choices for ourselves, whether it be having terrible relationships or work that makes a person miserable.
People with high self-esteem tend to have happier lives and demonstrate a higher quality of life.

3. A Greater Feeling of Inner Peace

Every person wants happiness and aspires to be happy, yet happiness is extremely interrelated with both physical and mental health. Mental health influences physical health, however the higher the amount of inner aggression, discord, and unpleasant emotions the poorer our mental health.

Negative psychological states such as distress, sadness, and anxiety have been shown connected with a greater risk of mental disease. Negative thoughts have been proven to have a crucial role in depression and psychological maladjustment.

One's optimistic ideas are discovered to be favorably associated with contentment with life and happiness. The wealthier we get in inner peace, the healthier our mind becomes. This sensation of completeness and realignment of mind and body, combined with a sense of inner harmony, is frequently mirrored in the spiritual and wisdom.

Mental tranquility is more about being than doing. It's about leaning towards rather than straining against.

It's about being totally present and focused on the work at hand. The blessings of inner serenity are countless. They include mental and physical health and well-being, self-confidence, stronger relationships, and a more passionate and happy experience in life.

Most of us desire these things, but sometimes we must reallocate our beliefs of ourselves and how we live in order to create an atmosphere that encourages inner calm. Once we make the adjustment, we must practice the acts that lead to inner calm in order to maintain it. The most crucial techniques to obtain peace of mind entail being honest with oneself, embracing the unpredictable nature of life, and observing one's thought process.

Many of us psychologically 'torture' ourselves by contemplating and obsessing over bad ideas which is really not a healthy habit instead we should examine our thoughts, pay less attention to the negative ones and concentrate on what we are grateful for in life.
 Practicing this frequently would undoubtedly pave the door for inner peace of mind.

Chapter 2.

Identifying signs of a troubled Mind.

Most people typically take serious warnings of poor mental health for granted. Such signals may be large or modest and may be discovered with diligent attention if mild.
The requirement for a steady mind cannot be over-emphasized! Basically, as living beings all our actions, and statements are first depicted in our brains before real projection, an unstable or wobbly mind consequently makes life a living hell
As noted previously the indicators of failing mental health may be mild or serious. Some of them include:

FEELING IRRITABLE

Everyone feels upset from time to time, but repeated feelings of irritation might suggest a larger issue. If you find yourself lashing out at individuals around you or being troubled by trivial matters, it may be time to take a step back and check on your general mental health.

PROBLEMS SLEEPING

Sleep is necessary for everyone, but it is particularly critical for people in recovery. Getting adequate sleep offers you the energy required to make it through the day and keeps your attitude up. If you are having chronic sleep issues such as sleeping too much or sleeping too little, you may be suffering from depression or anxiety symptoms.

CONSTANT FEELINGS OF DEPRESSION

Feeling sad is a natural feeling, but it becomes abnormal when you experience it most of the time. Depression may express itself in numerous ways, such as a lack of interest in once-loved hobbies, having low energy, or feeling sad all the time. If you have frequent emotions of sorrow that you can't seem to escape, it may be an indication your mental health is deteriorating.

FEELING DISCONNECTED FROM REALITY

When you are suffering, it might be easy to let your thoughts consume you whole.

You may feel as if you are living in an altogether separate universe from others, leading you to feel detached from not just the people around you but from the actual reality, you are in. Feeling this attitude might be harmful since it may lead you into undesirable activities that you wouldn't normally engage in.

ISOLATING FROM FRIENDS AND FAMILY

Taking time for yourself is vital from time to time, but isolating yourself and ignoring friends and family might suggest a problem. It is vital to have social interaction, as it may raise your mood and prevent getting eaten by inner, intrusive thoughts.

PROBLEMS CONCENTRATING

Those who deal with poor mental health frequently find themselves performing badly at school or jobs because they cannot focus on even the slightest of tasks. The poor focus has to do with the brain shifting into survival mode and devoting energy towards tasks that keep the individual alive rather than other critical duties.

CHANGES IN WEIGHT OR APPETITE

If you have witnessed a rapid rise or loss of weight, declining mental health may be the explanation.
Many people use food as a strategy for coping. Other folks overeat, while other people lose their appetite, culminating in dramatic weight changes.

PERSISTENT FEELINGS OF GUILT

Intrusive thoughts that cause you disproportionate feelings of guilt could be a symptom of poor mental health. You may be having thoughts such as, "I'm a failure," "No one will ever love me," or "Everything is my fault." You may even begin to indulge in self-degrading acts such as frequently making jokes about how horrible you are or always taking the blame for things. Bad mental health could cause you to feel guilty for numerous reasons, resulting in this self-deprecating humor and intrusive thoughts.

POOR PERSONAL HYGIENE

When you have poor mental health, it is normal to go into survival mode, which is focusing your attention on things that keep you alive, such as eating, drinking water, and sleeping. Things like hygiene are put on the back burner since you won't have the energy for them. These feelings may lead to less frequent washing, tooth cleaning, and hair combing.

Others may label you as lethargic when, in reality, you just lack the energy to commit to these pursuits.

SUICIDAL THOUGHTS

Suicide is a major health hazard, with the worldwide suicide death rate equivalent to 1.4% of all fatalities globally.

Most suicides are connected to mental illness, with depression, drug use disorders, and psychosis being the most prominent risk factors. However, anxiety, personality-, eating-, and trauma-related diseases, as well as basic mental abnormalities, all contribute.

A psychological autopsy from the middle of the previous century and onward have indicated that most individuals who have died by suicide had suffered from mental issues. A recent study reveals this number may be as least 90%. On the other hand, most folks with mental issues do not die by their own hand. The chance of suicide has been estimated to be 5–8% for several mental illnesses, such as depression, alcoholism, and schizophrenia

A stress-diathesis model has been created in which the risk for suicide acts is impacted not only by a mental state (the stressor) but also by a diathesis, such as a propensity to have higher suicidal thoughts and to be more willing to act on suicidal sentiments. Thus, suicide risk is multi-factorial.

Note: Please if you observe any of the aforementioned signs, backing down on the battle for your own peace of mind is not an option!!

Chapter 3
Utilitzing your spiritual resources.

Your journey to mental redemption starts from this very chapter. Endeavor to read with keen understanding.

Just the way physical health is dependent on your state of mind so is one's soul and mind...Yes... The Mind and soul are very much connected; the projection of one's soul depends on one's state of mind. One's mental state is often confused with one's soul, these two entities are entirely different but highly connected just like an unborn child and a mother, but still, differences exist.

Let us uncover the difference between the mind and soul and hence, look at how spirituality affects our mental wellness.

What difference between one's mind and soul?

Mind is only a representation of spirit. The soul is your full awareness, the living energy in you. The part of it which is listening to me right now is asking the question, which is perceiving - we call it the mind.
So if your mind is elsewhere, despite I'm speaking and the words are coming into your eardrums, nevertheless you don't grasp it because the mind is elsewhere.

So it's via the mind that we see, smell, taste, hear, and feel the sensation of touch. That is what the mind is.

The mind has another function which we call intelligence. As I'm speaking, something in you is saying, "Yes, I agree", or, "No, I don't agree with this". There is something in you that is accepting and rejecting, judging and adapting – that is intelligence. There is something in you that doesn't change, which is the reference point for all changes. Your ideas are changing, your emotions are changing, and your body has endured so much change. If you look at a 32 year ago an image of you, you can't swear it's the same body.

It's a lot different from what you are today, yet nonetheless, you are the same person. Something in you doesn't change. That non-changing part in you, or the reference by which you identify the changes so to say 'this is changing, there should be something that doesn't change, and that is what is the soul.

How one's Spirituality affects mental well-being?

The notion of spirituality signifies various things for different individuals. The range of spiritual beliefs and rituals is as diverse as the individuals who follow them.
One thing they all have in common is the breadth of effects they may have on our mental health.

Spirituality influences our mental health in a number of ways. Spirituality is your belief or feeling of purpose and meaning. It is what gives you a feeling of value or worth in your life. Contrary to what many people would assume, spirituality and religion are not the same. But they are related. You may be spiritual without adhering to a certain faith. Religious persons follow a particular religion and may be affiliated with certain organizations or traditions.

Impact of Spirituality on Mental Health

Spirituality impacts many choices that humans make. It promotes individuals to develop better connections with themselves, others, and the unknown.

Spirituality may help you cope with stress by providing you with a feeling of serenity, purpose, and forgiveness. It typically becomes more crucial in times of emotional stress or disease.

Positive impacts of spirituality. There are various ways that spirituality might assist your mental health:

· You may experience a greater sense of purpose, tranquillity, optimism, and significance.

· You may enjoy improved confidence, self-esteem, and self-control.

· It may help you make sense of your events in life.

· When ailing, it may help you experience inner strength and result in a speedier recovery.

· Those in a spiritual group may have greater assistance.
· You may work towards improved connections with yourself and others. Many persons with mental conditions obtain a feeling of optimism by conversing with a religious or spiritual leader. Some mental diseases might be understood as moments when individuals doubt their worth or purpose in a manner that leaves them feeling depressed. It may be tremendously useful to integrate spirituality into the therapy of mental health concerns.

What exactly are "spiritual resources"?

Spiritual resources are activities, beliefs, artifacts, or connections that individuals commonly turn to for aid in times of crisis or distress.

Some spiritual resources include:

- *Music*

Listening to music may be fun, and some study shows that it could even make you healthier. Music may be a source of joy and satisfaction, but there are many more psychological advantages as well

Music may ease the mind, revitalize the body, and even help individuals better manage pain.

The concept that music may impact your thoughts, emotions, and behavior probably does not come as much of a surprise. If you've ever been pumped up while listening to your favorite fast-paced rock song or been brought to tears by a delicate live performance, then you readily comprehend the power of music to affect emotions and even motivate action.

The psychological impacts of music may be profound and wide-ranging. Music therapy is an intervention occasionally used to enhance mental health, assist patients to deal with stress, and increase psychological well-being. Some studies even imply that your choice of music might give insight into various areas of your personality.

Music is an essential aspect of daily life and plays a major role in all human cultures: it is pervasive and is listened to and performed by humans of all ages, races, and ethnic origins. But music is not merely entertainment: a scientific study has proven that it may alter physiological processes that increase physical and mental wellness.

Music and Mental Health: The Science

The study surrounding how music affects our thoughts informs us that music stimulates our brains in a way that nothing else does. Researchers have noticed how, while gazing at a person listening to music in an MRI scanner, the brain lights up in a very unique manner.

Our brains are responsive to music and maybe that means we experience its advantages in a wide variety of diverse ways.

Music causes the production of neurochemicals that may assist increase our mental wellbeing.

When we listen to or play music, our brains produce dopamine, often known as the happy hormone, that we connect with pleasure and reward as well as serotonin, which is our bodies' natural mood stabilizer.

Listening to music, particularly music paired with nature sounds, has been demonstrated to reduce levels of cortisol which is a stress hormone that may naturally lessen anxiety and tension.

Whilst listening to music before a stressful event doesn't stop your cortisol levels from increasing when the event happens, listening to music after a stressful event may help you recover quicker. Music therapy has also been proven to raise levels of oxytocin, a hormone that the brain generates that improves our capacity to connect with others.

For these reasons, music has become a significant aspect of several mental health treatments because of its capacity to assist treat those battling sadness, anxiety, schizophrenia, and even dementia.

Here are five tips on how to use music to benefit your mental health in a practical way.

1. Relaxation

Because music may be so beneficial in relaxing after a high-stress day, it can be a terrific tool for meditation and mindfulness. Meditation seems severe, but is only the discipline of self-reflection, of allowing yourself some time every day to check in with your feelings. It may be done with a simple breathing technique that is aimed to decrease your heart rate, reduce stress and anxiety, and/or minimize panic attacks.

2. Motivation

Having a solid fitness regimen is a pretty crucial aspect of controlling your mental health. It may be getting up and doing some simple stretches, it might be going for a run or a stroll in the sunlight. Whatever it is, sometimes we might struggle to get moving, particularly if we are feeling depressed. Music may be a terrific method to get us moving. Choose your greatest encouragement tune and start going! The mix of music and movement can enhance your dopamine and serotonin levels and have you feeling brighter and more alert in no time!

3. Stimulation

Music may be particularly effective for providing you with a burst of energy when you are battling low mood, depression, lethargy, or exhaustion. Sometimes, it may be very helpful to slam on a piece of fantastic music and throw yourself a three-minute dance party, to give your head a nice rush of dopamine and make you feel a bit better! Or, alternatively, maybe you need to throw on a hard metal song and have a good old scream to relieve some of that stress! Stimulating your thoughts with music and giving yourself a surge of hormones will help you feel more invigorated.

4. Creation

Not everyone can be a composer or a musician, but practically everyone has a song that they genuinely feel 'speaks' to them and gives voice to their thoughts within. This might be especially beneficial if you are difficult to articulate your feelings. You may jot down song lyrics and use them as a starting point for some journaling. Don't worry about what you are writing or evaluate it on whether it is 'good' or not, just put down precisely how these music lyrics connect to you.

This creative process may be incredibly fulfilling and comforting when we are feeling overwhelmed or like our heads are too 'full.'

5. Elation

Music may offer pleasure. It may be community and pleasure and enthusiasm. Music is also strongly tied to memory, so harness that. Play songs that are tied to wonderful memories, share them with others in your life and utilize those happy memories to raise your mood. Enjoy the music that you love and derive delight from it!

Effects of Music On Managing Pain

Research has revealed that music may be highly useful in the treatment of pain. One research of fibromyalgia patients revealed that those who listened to music for only one hour a day saw a substantial decrease in pain compared to those in a control group.

At the conclusion of the four-week trial period, those who had listened to music each day showed substantial decreases in feelings of pain and despair. Such findings show that music therapy might be an essential technique in the treatment of chronic pain.

A 2015 review of studies on the impact of music on pain management indicated that patients who listened to music before, during, or even after surgery had less pain and worries than people who did not listen to music.

While listening to music at any point in time was useful, the researchers found that listening to music pre-surgery resulted in superior results.

The analysis looked at data from more than 7,000 patients and found that music listeners also needed less medicine to control their pain. There was also a somewhat higher, but not statistically significant, increase in pain management outcomes when patients were permitted to pick their own music.

The effects of music on one's mental state cannot be over-emphasized making music "One of The Most Powerful Tools In Combating Mental Decline". It is imperative we treat Music as a very powerful spiritual resource.

- *Prayer*

What is prayer?

Prayer has a highly particular meaning stemming from an individual's religious background or spiritual practice. For some, prayer will imply precise holy words; for others, it may be a more casual talking or listening to God or a higher force.

The term "prayer" derives from the Latin precarious, which means "obtained by pleading, to implore." Prayer is built on the concept that there is a force larger than oneself that may impact one's life. It is the act of lifting hearts and minds to God or a higher force.

There is no one specific manner to pray. Forms include verbal prayers, quiet prayers, and prayers of the thought, the heart, and oneness with God. Prayers may be directed (e.g., prayers for particular items) or non-directed, having no specific goal in mind.

The Neuroscience Behind Prayer. Serotonin is recognized by many experts as the "happy" neurotransmitter since it is crucial to helping to carry impulses from one section of the brain to another. Another function of serotonin is how it affects our mood and adds to our general feeling of wellness.

Research has proven that prayer has a direct influence on the brain's creation of serotonin and bathes the neurons in the chemical enriching lives and melting away tension. Indeed, prayer has a replenishing impact on serotonin and other vital neurotransmitters to produce an environment where new brain cells are formed and making individuals who practice it happier and healthier. It may also be suggested that serotonin isn't simply stimulated by prayer but that it is accountable for religiosity in people entire. Research undertaken by Borg, Bengt, et al. (2003) discovered a link between the serotonin system in normal male individuals was a foundation for religious experiences.

• *Meditation/Yoga*
What Does It Mean to Meditate?
What Is Meditation?

The word "meditation" refers to a collection of practices that one might utilize to obtain a heightened level of awareness and enhanced concentration. Because of this, it might be challenging to define meditation.

There are many different techniques to meditate. Most people assume that meditation always requires sitting cross-legged on a cushion with the eyes closed. Some even envision chanting mingled in.

This is one example, but there are many various styles of meditation that one may practice, including standing or walking meditations.

Is Meditation a Good Way to Improve Mental Health?

Meditation may assist people to lessen their sympathetic nervous system activity. This is also recognized as their "fight or flight" reaction. As a consequence, people feel calmer and more at ease, particularly during stressful circumstances.

People with depression and anxiety tend to have issues with intrusive, distracting thoughts.

Because of this, these thoughts may swiftly rise into major fears or regrets regarding the past.

Meditation makes it simpler for them to be in the present moment and avoid obsessing over these ideas.

How to Meditate?

Meditation is easier than most people imagine. Read these instructions, make sure you're someplace where you can relax into this process, set a timer, and give it a shot:

1) Take a seat

Findspot to sit that seems serene and quiet to you.

2) Set a time restriction

If you're just starting, it might assist to set a small duration, such as five or 10 minutes.

3) Notice your body

You can sit in a chair with your feet on the floor, you can sit loosely cross-legged, you may kneel—all are good. Just make sure you are steady and in a position, you can remain in for a long.

4) Feel your breath

Follow the feeling of your breath as it goes in and as it goes out.

5) Notice when your attention has drifted

Inevitably, your focus will leave the breath and move to other locations. When you come around to detecting that your mind has wandered—in a few seconds, a minute, five minutes—simply restore your focus to the breath.

6) Be compassionate to your wandering thoughts

Don't condemn yourself or stress about the substance of the ideas you find yourself caught in. Just come back.

7) Close with kindness

When you're ready, gradually elevate your gaze (if your eyes are closed, open them) (if your eyes are closed, open them). Take a minute and observe any noises in the area. Notice how your body feels right now.
Notice your ideas and feelings.
That's it! That's the practice. You concentrate your attention, your mind wanders, you bring it back, and you attempt to do it as sweetly as possible (as many times as you need to) (as many times as you need to).

How Much Should I Meditate?

Meditation is no more complex than I've stated before. It is that easy … and that tough. It's also strong and worth it.

The goal is to resolve to sit every day, even if it's for five minutes. One of my meditation instructors mentioned that the most crucial time in your meditation practice is the moment you sit down to do it. Because right then you're declaring to yourself that you believe in change, you believe in caring for yourself, and you're making it true. You're not simply retaining some value like mindfulness or compassion in the abstract, but genuinely making it real.

A recent study from many neuroscientists suggests that 12 minutes of meditation, 5 days a week may safeguard and develop your capacity to pay attention and as well boost your mental wellness.

Yoga is performed by more than 36 million Americans and by many millions more globally. A practice that is thousands of years old, yoga has spiritual and intellectual foundations. Many who practice it, particularly in the U.S., want physical advantages. There are also tremendous advantages of yoga for your mental wellness.

A sharper brain

When you lift weights, your muscles develop stronger and larger.
When you practice yoga, your brain cells establish new connections, and changes occur in brain structure as well as function, resulting in better cognitive abilities, such as learning and memory.

Yoga enhances areas of the brain that play a major role in memory, attention, consciousness, cognition, and language. See it as an exercise for the brain.

Studies using MRI scans and other brain imaging technology have shown that people who regularly did yoga had a thicker cerebral cortex (the location of the brain responsible for processing information) and hippocampus (the pace of the mind responsible for memory and learning) compared with non-practitioners. These parts of the brain generally decrease as you age, but the older yoga practitioners exhibited less shrinkage than those who practiced no yoga. This implies that yoga may offset age-related losses in memory and other cognitive functions.

Benefits of Yoga for Mental Health

There are many kinds of yoga. The type most practiced in the U.S. is the hatha yoga, that constitutes both mindful breathing and physical poses. Yoga can improve balance, flexibility, range of motion, and strength.

It also enhances one's mental well-being. According to many studies, yoga can:

Release helpful brain chemicals: Most exercise causes the production of "feel-good" neurotransmitters in the brain. These mood-enhancing compounds include brain messengers such as dopamine, serotonin, and norepinephrine.

Although yoga motions are calm and regulated, they nonetheless boost your heart rate, make the muscles work hard, and trigger the release of brain chemicals. As a consequence, yoga may make you happy.

Relieve depression:
Studies suggest that yoga helps relieve depression. Researchers have shown that yoga is equivalent to other therapies, such as medicine and psychotherapy.
Yoga is frequently affordable and doesn't have the same negative effects as many drugs. It may even aid persons with the significant depressive condition. The use of yoga for depression requires additional investigation since there aren't too many controlled studies.

Reduced stress:

When Americans completed a study on why they practiced yoga, 86% of them indicated that it helps them cope with stress. The tightening and relaxation of muscles may relieve stress. You may also benefit from the tranquil ambiance, relaxing music, and positive attitude that you will find in most yoga programs.

Ease anxiousness:

Yoga may alleviate anxiety. The breath training contained in yoga may be particularly useful, given there is a link between nervousness and breathing issues. If you have been diagnosed with an anxiety illness, yoga may not help. Still, some psychologists are utilizing yoga to enhance other types of treatment.

Improve sleep:
Research shows that yoga might enhance sleep. This may be particularly true for elderly folks. In one research of yoga practitioners over the age of 60, individuals reported an improvement in both the quality and quantity of their sleep. They also raised their sleep efficiency, which assesses the proportion of time in bed actually spent sleeping.

Enhance social life:
 If you attend an in-person yoga session, you may benefit from socializing with others in your group. Social bonds may favorably improve both mental and physical health.

Also, behaving in conjunction with others, commonly termed synchronization, has special social advantages. Moving and breathing at the same time as others might give you a feeling of belonging and foster a connection with the group.

Promotes other good practices: If you practice yoga, you may be more inclined to pick more healthful meals. Yoga may also be a doorway to other sorts of physical exercise. Exposure to other health-minded individuals might motivate you to adopt additional healthy lifestyle choices.

Besides these advantages, yoga may be good for persons seeking to reduce weight, quit smoking, and manage chronic illness. Of course, your outcomes may vary.

Your success might rely upon your mind set, the quality of your education, and the sort of yoga being done.

Using Yoga to Improve Your Mental Health

The ideal approach to learning yoga is with a certified instructor, either in an individual session or in a group. A yoga instructor may correct your positions and show you how to alter them if required. You may use blocks, belts, and other materials to make certain positions simpler.

You can even practice yoga on a chair instead of on the floor.

It's also feasible to learn yoga online or via a book or DVD. But the best method to prevent damage is to join an in-person yoga session.

Once you get the fundamentals down, you may utilize books and videos to help you practice. You will gain more from yoga if you practice it at home between courses, and online programs may keep your home practice exciting. If you are comfortable performing yoga at home, you may practice it when you suffer excessive stress, insomnia, or other issues.

- ***Church, and social support groups***

Spirituality and religion can give a feeling of comfort and social structure and those beliefs may be a great coping tool during tough circumstances. Being an active part of a close-knit religious group may give structure, support, and a feeling of acceptability, all of which are helpful to mental health. The connectivity of a group may make members feel welcomed and respected. There are also specific life conditions or occurrences that might question religious ties and beliefs. This might include chronic disease, death of a loved one, or simply feelings of rejection during times of transition.

It's at these challenging moments that people may seek outside of their religious group or trusted spiritual leaders for direction on how to handle the circumstance and retain mental well-being.

The Concept of A Support Group

A support group is a meeting of individuals experiencing similar challenges to communicate what's upsetting them. Through the sharing of experiences, they're able to give support, encouragement, and comfort to the other group members, and get the same in return.

When you're going through a tough or distressing moment, family members and friends may empathize, but they don't always know what to say or the best methods to assist.

Doctors and health professionals may occasionally give little emotional assistance, but their main emphasis is always medical.

Support groups are designed to unite individuals together who are suffering from similar challenging situations. That may be dealing with a particular medical illness, such as cancer or dementia, a mental health issue like depression, anxiety, grief, or addiction, for example, or caring for a family member or friend confronting such a problem. Whatever troubles you or a loved one are suffering, however, the greatest medication might sometimes be the voice of individuals who have walked in your shoes.

A support group gives a secure location where you may acquire knowledge that's practical, constructive, and beneficial. You'll have the advantage of encouragement, and you'll learn more about dealing with your challenges via shared experiences. Hearing from people having similar issues might sometimes help you feel less alone in your struggles.

Benefits of support groups

A support group is a secure environment where you may speak about your feelings and situations with people who know how you feel and won't judge or condemn you. It may also assist you to:

Learn better-coping methods.

As you go through hard conditions, you may need to find new strategies to deal with. At a support group, you'll learn coping methods from others who've found success using them first-hand. You could discover tips on meditating, writing, or topics you wouldn't have otherwise considered. You could also pick up new techniques to create healthy limits and operate better.

Grow via shared experiences.

A support group provides you an opportunity to get things off your chest. Sharing your personal experiences with the group might help relieve your emotional weight and feelings of loneliness.

As individuals in the group share their tales, you might receive vital information about how others cope with similar challenges.

Focus on self-care.
Support group members may give up unique suggestions for how to care for themselves, handle stress, overcome weariness, and feel mentally and physically stronger.

Maintain a feeling of hope.
Being with your fellow support group members may help increase your mood and feeling of hope, providing you the emotional reserves to genuinely picture a brighter future.

- ***Inspirational writings***
  - *Poetry; as a case study.*

Poetry Therapy

Poetry therapy, a sort of expressive arts therapy, includes the therapeutic use of poems, narratives, and other spoken or written media to promote well-being and healing. Therapists may utilize current literature as part of treatment or inspire persons in therapy to generate their own literary works to communicate deep-seated feelings.

In any instance, they provide a secure, non-judgmental setting in which persons in therapy are allowed to examine their written expressions and related emotional reactions.

Benefits of Poetry
Improves creative thinking and blasts stress:

While composing poetry you need to wrack your thoughts and focus on metaphors and pictures. Writing poetry may assist cultivate and enhance creative thinking. You get more creative and begin to think more and more which is a terrific workout for your brain and helps distract your attention from other awful events in life which in turn helps you fight stress.

Helps relieve emotional pain:

Whether it is postpartum sadness or any type of unpleasant feeling you are going through, writing poetry expressing the agony helps you vent out your suffering and consequently makes you feel better. Many of the world's most inspiring poetries have portrayed grief in the most beautiful manner. Memorializing or paying homage to individuals you've lost makes you feel better and helps you forget your regret.

Helps boost cognitive function:
The stages involved in creating a poem, right from seeking the correct word or structuring the sentences, or fine-tuning the rhythm of a poem help develops your cognitive skills.

Helps develop self-awareness:
Poetry writing helps you discover yourself and see your inner reflection. What you are drawn to or do you enjoy writing about? It offers you an optimistic view of life.

Unstable emotions or indecisiveness may affect your mental serenity. And after you finish composing a piece of poetry, you see a bit of you in it.

These materials(Spiritual Resources) may help individuals return to a feeling of equilibrium after their lives have been flipped upside down. They can assist individuals sort through the "big" issues in order to discover meaning, comfort, hope, kindness, and community in the face of a catastrophe.

Your own unique spiritual resource(s) may not be discovered in this chapter; simply explore your inner self and see what you are intimately linked to. Such a strong connection if any is clearly a sign pointing in the direction of your spiritual resource. Hold onto it and maximize it; making you into your greatest version!

Chapter 4
Voicing out helps.

Seeking assistance is crucial and should never be stigmatized!!

Seeking treatment is frequently the first step towards becoming and staying well, but talking about a mental health condition isn't always easy. It's natural to feel uncomfortable about speaking about your health to a trusted friend or family member - and asking your doctor or workplace for support might seem daunting.

Talking to people about feelings, emotions, and ideas may help your mental health.

Many individuals may believe that talking to others might produce a sense of weakness, although talking to others can lower stress and enhance health. Communicating with others may help you feel supported and provide people the capacity to sympathize and give you advice.
By speaking out, you'll contribute to eradicating the stigma around ailments like anxiety and depression. At the same time, you'll make sure that you find the proper degree of care and social support that you require.

Why it's vital to reach out?
It's vital to reach out when you are coping with mental health difficulties.

This could include anything from suicidal thoughts to feelings of loneliness or anxiety.

Even if you don't think that reaching out would change anything, it's still necessary to do so.

By reaching out and being honest about what you are going through, you're more likely to receive the correct guidance and support you need.

Every individual who seeks treatment also contributes to the decline of stigmas related to mental health. This will make it simpler for future assistance seekers to locate the direction they desire.

It's not always feasible to reach out knowing precisely what you need from others.

However, merely declaring that you don't want to be alone notifies the people around you that you need more attention and assistance at a given moment.

It also alerts them to the idea that they may need to aid you in obtaining treatment.

Who to Talk To About Your Mental Health With?

Opening up about your mental troubles can enable you to communicate how you genuinely feel and it provides others an opportunity to support you by guiding you through the tough periods. You may speak about your concerns with a trustworthy family member, friend, mentor, or therapist.

Bottling up these ideas might eventually evolve into a greater problem. It is of tremendous importance if you chat with someone you can entrust; depend on to be proactive about your existing status. Conveying Your Message To Someone

Make a Plan

Before you sit down with a loved one or a therapist to inform them about your diagnosis, consider these tips:
Set the tone. Frame the discussion so your friend, loved one, or co-worker knows that what you're going to say is different from your regular chitchat. Say something like, "I'd want to talk to you about something important.

I'm hoping you'll be patient and make an effort to comprehend. It's hard for me to discuss personal things."
Be specific. If your disclosure includes a plea for aid, make clear precisely what you need: Can you help me locate a therapist? Would you transport me to appointments? Sometimes I become anxious: Can I call you?

The advantages of obtaining assistance

Actively seeking psychiatric therapy has several immediate and long-term advantages, including:

1. You will no longer suffer alone

Dealing with a mental disease may be an immensely isolated experience.

And battling alone isn't the way to getting through terrible circumstances.

Seeking assistance guarantees that you may establish a support group that understands what you're going through. This community may give useful and suitable suggestions and assistance.

2. You can create better connections

Mental health therapy can enable you to reconnect with your loved ones. You'll establish stronger, healthier relationships via straightforward and honest communication.

3. It minimizes your chances for various medical conditions

Poor mental health might also create other physiological difficulties. Poor sleep and sleep disorders, obesity, digestive issues, and other ailments are all connected. Seeking care early on can lessen your chances of acquiring additional health concerns.

4. It teaches you to create coping methods

Seeking professional therapy will offer you the coping techniques and tactics you need. You'll be able to negotiate hard circumstances with a higher degree of awareness.

5. Your performance at work may increase

Mental health disorders might negatively impair our job performance.

They have the power to make us demotivated and dejected. Seeking assistance enables you to learn how to handle issues that might influence your well-being and mental health. You'll perform to the best of your abilities, even when you are under pressure

6. It increases your quality of life

Acquiring support can assist you in developing your connections and making new acquaintances.

You'll also learn how to handle obstacles that arise on a regular basis

while identifying what does and doesn't work for you.
All of these things may positively affect your life in the long term while generating a healthier and happier you.

Chapter 5
Popular Questions Regarding Mental Health.

The issue of mental health is no longer taboo, and more of us are entering the dialogue. But many of us still have questions…

1. What is a personality disorder?

If you have been diagnosed with a personality disorder it doesn't imply that you're fundamentally different from everyone else, although at times you may require special help.

The term 'personality' refers to the pattern of thoughts, emotions, and conduct that makes each of us the people that we are.

These impact the way we think, feel and behave towards others and ourselves.

We don't always think, feel and react in precisely the same way - it depends on the circumstances we are in, the people around us, and many other variables. But we typically tend to act in rather predictable ways.

Personality disorders are a sort of mental health condition when your attitudes, beliefs, and actions give you ongoing troubles in your life.

You alone have a unique experience with personality disorder. However, you could regularly have problems with how you see other people and yourself. It could be difficult for you to change these undesirable behaviors.

2. What is post-traumatic stress disorder (PTSD)?

The term PTSD is used to describe a variety of psychological symptoms, which may follow traumatic experiences. PTSD may be triggered by anything that consciously, or subconsciously, reminds a person of a particular incident in their life. For some individuals, this is a single, huge, momentous incident – such as a car accident – and for others a continuing sequence of occurrences, such as being in combat zones, or facing abuse.

Symptoms of PTSD don't generally manifest immediately away, and in others, don't develop until several years after the occurrence.

They might include intense memories, nightmares, difficulty of sleep, and feeling emotionally cut off. PTSD is surprisingly widespread - as many as 10% of the population may experience it at some point in their life.

If someone has been living with unpleasant symptoms for over a month following a traumatic experience they should contact their GP, who can refer them for specialized care. Effective therapy does exist, and you can recover from PTSD.

3. Are drugs or therapy better for mental health conditions?

Different individuals will discover that different treatments assist to manage their mental health - whether this is medication, or alternatives such as talking therapy, exercise, or a blend.

While antidepressants may be useful for some, they are not the answer for everyone and are not typically advised as first-line therapy for mild to severe depression. Anyone using antidepressants should be made aware of the prospective positives and drawbacks for them, and they should have their therapy reassessed often.

Talking treatments such as cognitive behavioral therapy (CBT) and counseling are becoming more widely offered as part of the Improving

Access to Psychological Therapies project. Giving individuals a choice of treatments is crucial, whether that's medications, talking therapies, or alternatives such as art therapy or exercise.

4. How can I speak to and help someone with a mental health problem like depression or anxiety?

Here are some thoughts on how you may support folks struggling with anxiety and depression:

Encourage them to seek assistance

Perhaps the most essential thing you can do is urge them to get adequate therapy.

You may reassure them by letting them know that aid is out there and that you will be there to support them.

Don't be scared to bring it up

It takes a lot for someone to say, 'I need help, but it doesn't harm to address the issue yourself. Try to be upfront about depression and tough feelings, so kids know that it's OK to speak about what they're experiencing. Sometimes, you don't have to overtly discuss mental health to find out how they are doing — it may be as easy as contacting them to let them know you're thinking of them, or proposing that you go out for dinner or a stroll.

Don't blame them

Try not to criticize them for feeling nervous or sad, or advise them to 'pull themselves together.
They are undoubtedly already blaming themselves, and criticism is likely to make them feel much worse.

Exercise patience

Someone with depression may grow angrier, and be more inclined to misunderstand people, or feel misunderstood, than normal. They may require comfort in various instances.

Look after yourself

Your mental health is vital, too, and caring after someone else might place pressure on your wellness. If you are able to remain healthy, you are more likely to be able to give appropriate assistance for longer.

This might involve attempting to keep healthy and physically active, confiding in someone other than the person you are afraid about taking a vacation from time to time, and being realistic about what you can and can't accomplish yourself.

5. How can I know if someone has a mental health problem?

Common mental health conditions such as sadness and anxiety impact one in four persons. But it's still something that plenty of people find hard to speak about, which may mean that many individuals keep their thoughts about having a mental health condition a secret, even from close family and friends.

You can't always tell whether someone has a mental illness - individuals could seem as if they're OK and doing well, but in fact, they're quietly hurting.

If someone has a bipolar illness, they may display substantial mood fluctuations, or look more withdrawn if they are suffering from self-harm or negative thoughts, but everything is dependent on the person and there is no one method to identify whether someone is sick.

6. Is psychotherapy a replacement for medication?

Psychotherapy in certain situations might be adequate for the treatment of certain mental illnesses. However, it may be required in combination with medicines.

This is why in certain circumstances, it is not viewed as a replacement for medicine.

7. If a drug is recommended to me and I begin to feel better after taking it, is it alright to discontinue using it?

It is typical for individuals to stop taking their medicine when they believe their symptoms have gotten managed. Others may opt to cease their drug due to adverse effects. Another difficulty with taking medicine, particularly if you stop it suddenly, is that you may get withdrawal symptoms that may be quite unpleasant.

If your doctor believes you need to discontinue your prescription, it is vital to discuss it with your physician as he could be able to recommend another kind of medicine or change the amount of your medication.

8. What environmental factors influence mental illness?

Certain triggering situations, such as:
• Losses (physical loss after trauma, loss of important people, separation, etc...), might be severe stresses initiating a mental illness.
• Persistent dangers
• Prolonged exposure to distressing situations
• Negative family dynamics
• Extreme hardship and poverty
• Debilitating chronic disease and chronic pain
• Discrimination against minorities, for example

9. Why is it necessary for someone suffering from mental illness to follow a routine?

Mental illness may frequently interrupt a person's life by impairing that person's ability to concentrate on and accomplish things that they otherwise would be able to do. Establishing a productive daily pattern may assist to normalize that person's daily life and having a regular most typically helps to enhance life satisfaction that comes with personal success (in the human population as a whole, not just those living with mental illness) (in the human population as a whole, not just those living with mental illness).

10. Why do some individuals opt to only take drugs and no counseling, is it safe?

The choice to use prescription medicine is one that every person must decide for himself or herself. Some individuals may not feel comfortable giving information to physicians or others living with mental illness in a therapeutic atmosphere so they opt to depend exclusively on medicine to manage the disruptions in their life caused by mental disease.

The subject of whether it is safe to take prescription medicine without participation in treatment may best be addressed by noting that it could be less successful to take medication without the benefit of therapy.

It does not appear to have been demonstrated to be harmful.

11. What psychological factors can contribute to mental illness?

Psychological elements that may lead to mental illness include unique vulnerabilities such as personality characteristics, certain extremes in temperament features, a special sensitivity to unpleasant emotions, cognitive vulnerability, dysfunctional attitudes, despair, and negative distortions.

CONCLUSION

The concept of mental health cannot be over-looked. As days and years go by, people become more concerned about their physical state of being and pay little or no attention to the psychological factor of their health. One's mental health is like a power house, and without it, we most definitely cannot perform our daily tasks to the maximum. As much as we pay attention to our bodies, we should pay the same attention to our minds.

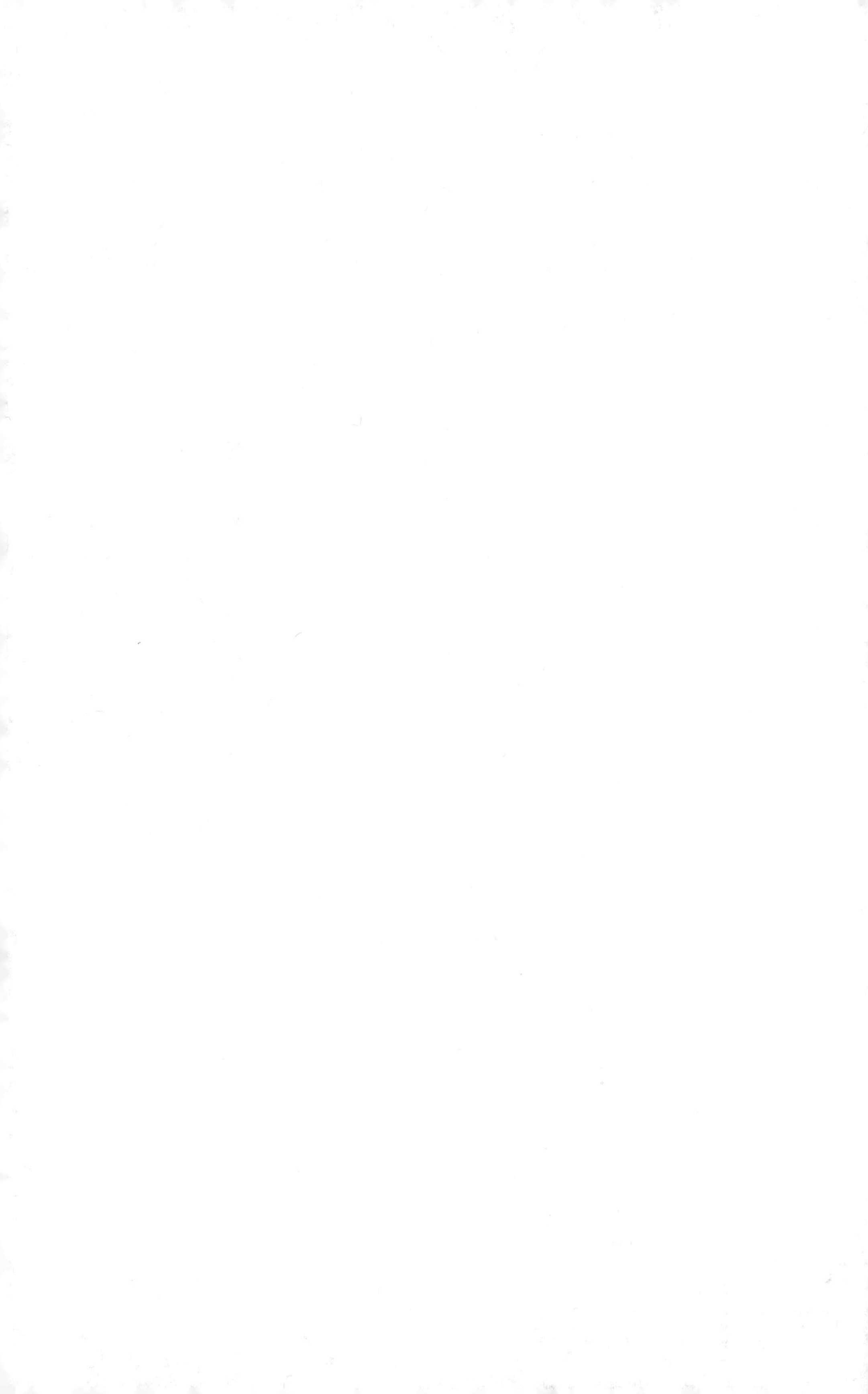

9 7983 5699 1233